Medical Education
Teaching and Learning Skills

Akmal El-Mazny

Copyright © 2016 Akmal El-Mazny

All rights reserved.

CreateSpace, Charleston SC, USA

ISBN-13: 978-1539012559
ISBN-10: 1539012557

Contents

	PAGE
Introduction	1
Evolution of Medical Education	2
Learning Cycle	3
Educational Objectives	4
Curriculum Design	6
Teaching Methodologies	11
– Teaching Large Groups	13
– Teaching Small Groups	22
– One to One Teaching	26
– Clinical Teaching	29
– Problem Based Learning (PBL)	42
– Web Based Learning	53
Learning Methodologies	59
Student Assessment	64
– Written Assessment	72
– Skill Based Assessment	74
– Work Based Assessment	78
Program Evaluation	79
Research in Medical Education	87
References	88

INTRODUCTION

Medical education is the science related to the practice of teaching and learning in medicine.

The ultimate aim of all stages of medical education - including basic medical education, postgraduate training, and continuing professional development - is to improve the medical care of the population.

By using teaching and learning methods based on educational theories and principles, medical educators will become more effective teachers.

This will enhance the development of knowledge, skills, and positive attitudes in their learners, and improve the next generation of teachers.

Eventually, this should result in better trained doctors who provide an even higher level of medical care and improved patient outcomes.

Everything is easy when you know how; this book has attempted to show how the gap between educational theory and practice can be bridged.

EVOLUTION OF MEDICAL EDUCATION

- "Most ideas about teaching are not new, but not everyone knows the old ideas" (Circa; 300 BC)
- Modern medical curricula design has been a struggle between the theory and the practice of medicine
- The model proposed by Flexner in the 1920s tried to strike a balance with 2 years of pre-clinical basic science training followed by 2-3 years of clinical training and was adopted by medical schools worldwide
- Flexnerian model has drawn criticisms for artificial separation of basic science and clinical practice
- Medical education has evolved to become more relevant for the changing needs of society and to adjust to the explosion of biomedical scientific knowledge
- Recent reforms in medical education includes greater emphasis on active and self-directed learning, across the board integration of disciplines, and generally a more humanistic and need-based approach to medical education

LEARNING CYCLE

- First: (1) Learning objectives and (2) Curriculum design
- Subsequently: (3) Teaching and (4) Learning methodologies
- Finally: (5) Student assessment and (6) Program evaluation

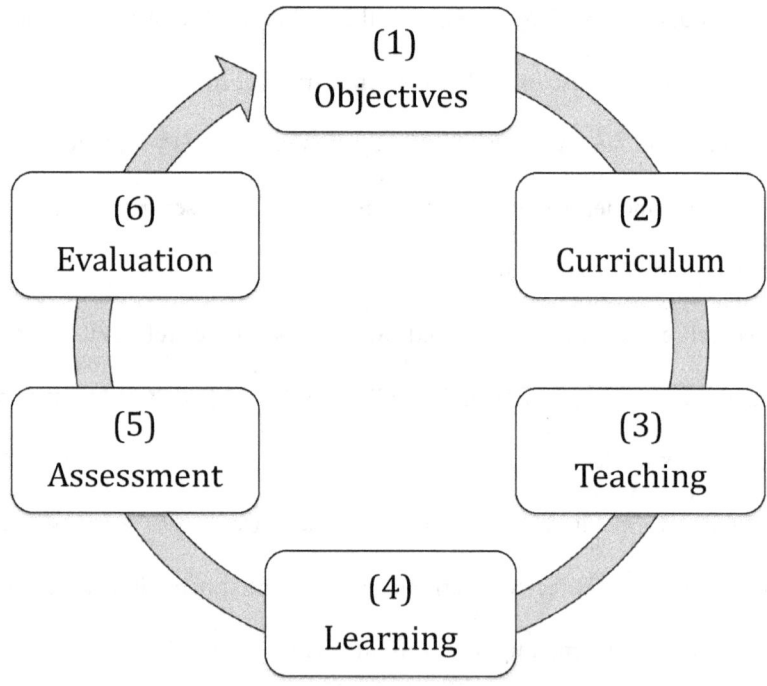

EDUCATIONAL OBJECTIVES

Classification of Educational Objectives

- Educational objectives are divided into three somewhat overlapping broad domains:

    (1) Cognitive (knowledge),

    (2) Psychomotor (skills), and

    (3) Affective (attitudes)

- Each of these domains are sub-classified into different levels that follow a hierarchical pattern
- The classification system is useful for many commonly performed educational activities such as developing learning objective, questioning during teaching, and assessment

Writing Educational Objectives

- Educational objectives are learner-centered, short, and precise descriptions of what learners are expected to achieve at the end of the program

- Good learning objectives include specifications about:

  (1) Target audience,

  (2) Observable/measurable behavior,

  (3) Conditions of learning, and

  (4) Degree of achievement

- Educational objectives are directly linked to teaching methods and assessment and evaluation

CURRICULUM DESIGN

Curriculum Planning

- Curriculum is a dynamic process that needs a systemic and stepwise implementation
- Curriculum should have a built-in feedback system with ample room for ongoing modification and adjustment
- Every curricular reform faces a predictable pattern of resistance
- A broad-based consensus among the faculty members is crucial for successful implementation
- Support from the dean and the students has very valuable impact on the reform process
- Clearly stated objectives provide a good starting point, but behavioural objectives are no longer accepted as the "gold standard" in curriculum design

Levels of Curriculum

The Planned Curriculum

– What is intended by the designers

The Delivered Curriculum

– What is organised by the administrators

– What is taught by the teachers

The Experienced Curriculum

– What is learned by the students

Curriculum Models

Prescriptive Model

– What curriculum designers should do

– How to create a curriculum

Descriptive Model

– What curriculum designers actually do

– What a curriculum covers

Objectives Model

– What educational purposes should the institution seek to attain

– What educational experiences are likely to attain the purposes

– How can these educational experiences be organised effectively

– How can we determine whether these purposes are being attained

Behavioural Objectives

Acceptable Verbs	Unacceptable Verbs
−To write	−To know
−To recite	−To understand
−To identify	−To really understand
−To differentiate	−To appreciate
−To solve	−To fully appreciate
−To construct	−To grasp the significance of
−To list	−To enjoy
−To compare	−To believe
−To contrast	−To have faith in

Situational Analysis

External Factors

− Societal expectations and changes

− Expectations of employers

− Community assumptions and values

− Nature of subject disciplines

− Nature of support systems

− Expected flow of resources

Internal Factors

− Students

− Teachers

− Institutional ethos and structure

− Existing resources

− Problems and shortcomings in existing curriculum

TEACHING METHODOLOGIES

Competency in Medical Teaching

— Content competency is not enough to become an effective teacher

<u>Basic Competencies</u>

— Understanding and determination of application of learning concepts and philosophies

— Understanding the basics of curriculum planning and implementation

— Ability to plan and execute an educational program

— A competency in the range of teaching methodologies

— An ability to choose and administer proper assessment methods

<u>Major Innovations</u>

— Integrated and flexible curriculum models

— Problem-based and case-based leaning, greater use of small groups, role-play and other forms of collaborative and group learning

— Understanding of nature of medical expertise and clinical reasoning

— Development of assessment methods that are more valid and reliable for the intended purpose

Implementation of Teaching Methodologies

– There are many teaching methods which differ in their usefulness to achieve the demands of a particular task

– Traditional lecture and similar passive educational activities produce short-lived impact on the learners

– Transfer of learning into real-life improves progressively with active participation and practice

TEACHING LARGE GROUPS

Making Lecture Effective

– Lectures are still a common teaching method in both undergraduate and postgraduate medical education

– Their continued popularity is due to the fact that they represent an effective and efficient means of teaching new concepts and knowledge

– Lectures deliver a large amount of information to a sizeable number of audience

– A lecture is organized into basic sections of:

(1) Introduction,

(2) Body, and

(3) Conclusion

Helping Students to Learn

− Use concrete examples to illustrate abstract principles

− Give handouts of the lecture slides, with space to write notes

− Give handouts with partially completed diagrams and lists for the students to complete during or after the lecture

− Allow for pauses in the delivery to give students time to write notes

− Check for understanding by asking questions or by running a mini-quiz

− Lack of active participation from the students is the major limitation of traditional lecture

− Lectures can be made interactive and participatory without jeopardizing the structure and cohesiveness with simple innovations such as questioning and periodic pause and review

Planning a Lecture

— How your lecture fits into the students' course or curriculum

— The students' knowledge of your subject; try to get a copy of the lecture and tutorial list for the course

— How the course (and your lecture) will be assessed

— The teaching methods that the students are accustomed to

Medium for Delivering the Lecture

- Which teaching media are available at the teaching venue
- Which teaching media are you familiar with (It is not always appropriate to experiment with new media)
- Which medium will best illustrate the concepts and themes that you want to teach the students
- Which medium would encourage students to learn through interaction during your lecture

Lecture Plan with a Classic Structure

– Outline purpose of lecture

– Describe main themes that will be covered

– Outline and explain first key point

– Illustrate with examples

– Repeat first key point

– Optional student activity to reinforce learning first key point

– Outline and explain second key point

– Illustrate with examples

– Repeat second key point

– Optional student activity to reinforce learning second key point

– Summarise

– Repeat main themes and conclude

Lecture Plan with a Problem Oriented Structure

– Statement of problem

– Offer solution 1

– Discuss strengths and weaknesses of solution 1

– Optional student activity based on solution 1

– Offer solution 2

– Discuss strengths and weaknesses of solution 2

– Optional student activity based on solution 2

– Summary and concluding remarks

Handouts

- Handouts can encourage better learning if they allow students more time to listen and think
- Handouts should provide a scaffold on which students can build their understanding of a topic
- Handouts should provide a summary of the major themes while avoiding an exhaustive explanation of each
- Handouts can be used to direct further learning, by including exercises and questions with suggested reading lists

Questioning Technique

- Good questioning is a major determinant of the success of teaching
- Justifying questions, clarification questions, hypothetical questions, and questions about the questions are better in promoting higher order thinking skill
- Failure of the student to respond to a particular question is often due to the lack of his understanding of the question
- A period of silence after a question is asked and after a response is given is essential

Effective Feedback

– Feedback is an educationally sound way of communicating teachers' observations to the students

– Feedback differs from criticism and praise and is more specific and descriptive

– The focus of feedback is behavior change and not judgement

– Feedback in group situations should include soliciting self-assessment and self-suggestion first

TEACHING SMALL GROUPS

Understanding Small Group

- Small group is formed when there are common learning goals
- Small group supports active and collaborative learning
- Variation in learning needs, style, and pace among the learners is a potential obstacle that needs to be overcome
- Group matures in identifiable phases: orientation, conflict, consensus, and closure
- An ideal group facilitates free exchange of ideas while remaining on target to fulfill the learning goals
- Tutors' responsibility in the group includes maintaining social organization and keeping the group on target

Problems Associated with Small Groups

– The teacher gives a lecture rather than conducting a dialogue

– The teacher talks too much

– Students cannot be encouraged to talk except with difficulty; they will not talk to each other, but will only respond to questions from the tutor

– Students do not prepare for the sessions

– One student dominates or blocks the discussion

– The students want to be given the solutions to problems rather than discuss them

Effective Facilitation in Small Group Discussion

−Ensure that group members have an agreed set of ground rules; for example, not talking at the same time as another group member

−Ensure that the students are clear about the tasks to be carried out

−When you present a question don't answer it yourself or try to reformulate it; count to 10 silently before speaking again

−When you have something you *could* say (which could be most of the time), count to 10 again

−Look round the group both when you are speaking and when a student is speaking; that way the students will quickly recognize that they are addressing the group rather than just you

Planning the Structure of a Small Group Discussion

Step 1

−Consider what you want the students to learn or achieve - in other words, what the learning outcomes should be

−For example, students will be able to identify and competently use three different general strategies for solving patients' problems

Step 2

−The group is given a problem to solve

−The students have to monitor the problem solving strategies that they are to use

−They then share their findings and compare them with research evidence

−They draw up a classification of the findings

Step 3

−Decide how to organise the small group

−Your tasks are to prepare any materials, explain and check agreement on the tasks, monitor the development of the tasks, and control time boundaries

ONE TO ONE TEACHING

Exceptional Potential of One to One Teaching

– It tackles current learning needs

– It promotes autonomy and self directed learning

– It links prior knowledge with new clinical experiences

– It enables opportunistic teaching

Monitor Progress

− Identify deficiencies

− Ask the learner, half way through the attachment, to do a self assessment of how things are going. If both you and the learner can identify deficiencies within a safe learning environment, you can work together to tackle them well before the attachment ends

− If you have serious concerns, you have an obligation to make them known to the learner and to the medical school or training authority

− It is not appropriate to diagnose serious problems and hand the learner on to the next stage of training in the hope that the problems will somehow be correct themselves

Promote Active Learning

- Wards, operating theatres, general practice, and community clinics provide a context for active learning
- Time is limited in most clinical settings, and it can be tempting to revert to a passive observational teaching model
- Think about strategies to promote active learning
- Brief students to observe specific features of a consultation or procedure
- Ask patients for permission for the learner to carry out all or part of the physical examination or a procedure while you observe
- If space is available, allow students to interview patients in a separate room or cubicle before presenting them to you
- If possible videotape consultations for a debriefing session at a more convenient time
- Arrange for the learner to see the same patient over time, or in another context, such as a home visit

CLINICAL TEACHING

Concepts and Rationale

- The educational characteristics of clinical teaching include patient-centeredness, encounter-specificity, unpredictability, promotion of clinical reasoning, and time constraints
- Precepting is analogous to social interaction that benefits from recognizing the other party's needs and expectations
- The successful preceptor has an interest in the learners' success
- The effective clinical teachers possess comprehensive knowledge base that goes beyond the knowledge of the subject matter

Delivery of Clinical Teaching

- "Microskill" model brings structure and logic in clinical teaching
- "Microskill" sequentially progresses from identifying learner's needs, providing general principles, and rendering feedback
- Promotion of clinical reasoning is an important goal of clinical teaching
- Each of the clinical reasoning process requires somewhat different teaching strategies
- Unusual patient stories, anecdotes and other clinical oddities may actually harm the learning process

Teaching Procedural Skills

- Procedural skills teaching involves comprehensive engagement of knowledge, attitude, and skill
- For teaching purposes, procedures are classified as:

    (1) Essential,

    (2) Elective, and

    (3) Not-required, not recommended

- Many conventional ways of teaching procedural skills are not scientifically sound
- Procedures can be taught in various ways depending upon the nature of procedures and students' own interest and ability
- Usual barriers for learning are lack of motivation, wrong image of the procedures, inherent inability, and difficulty of transferring skills to real situations

Teaching Communication Skills

- Good physician-patient communication improves patient related outcomes and benefits physicians
- Communication is a learnable and teachable skill
- Observation of "bedside manner" is an inefficient way of teaching communication skills
- Successful educational interventions require multi-pronged strategies including building up knowledge, demonstration, feedback, reflection, self-assessment, repeated practice in safe and simulated environment

Challenges of Clinical Teaching

—Time pressures

—Competing demands; clinical (especially when needs of patients and students conflict); administrative; research

—Often opportunistic; makes planning more difficult

—Increasing numbers of students

—Fewer patients (shorter hospital stays; patients too ill or frail; more patients refusing consent)

—Often under-resourced

—Clinical environment not "teaching friendly" (for example, hospital ward)

—Rewards and recognition for teachers poor

Common Problems with Clinical Teaching

- Lack of clear objectives and expectations

- Focus on factual recall rather than on development of problem solving skills and attitudes

- Teaching pitched at the wrong level (usually too high)

- Passive observation rather than active participation of learners

- Inadequate supervision and provision of feedback

- Little opportunity for reflection and discussion

- "Teaching by humiliation"

- Informed consent not sought from patients

- Lack of respect for privacy and dignity of patients

- Lack of congruence or continuity with the rest of the curriculum

Cognitive Learning Theory

− Help students to identify what they already know through brainstorming and briefing

− Provide a bridge between existing and new information; for example, use of clinical examples, comparisons, analogies

− Debrief the students afterwards

− Promote discussion and reflection

− Provide relevant but variable contexts for the learning

How to Use Questions

—Restrict use of closed questions to establishing facts or baseline knowledge (What? When? How many?)

—Use open or clarifying/probing questions in all other circumstances (What are the options? What if?)

—Allow adequate time for students to give a response; don't speak too soon

—Follow a poor answer with another question

—Resist the temptation to answer learners' questions; use counter questions instead

—Statements make good questions; for example, "students sometimes find this difficult to understand" instead of "Do you understand?" (which may be intimidating)

—Be non-confrontational; you don't need to be threatening to be challenging

How to Give Effective Explanations

− Check understanding before you start, as you proceed, and at the end; non-verbal cues may tell you all you need to know about someone's grasp of the topic

− Give information in "bite size" chunks

− Put things in a broader context when appropriate

− Summarise periodically ("so far, we've covered . . .") and at the end; asking learners to summarise is a powerful way of checking their understanding

− Reiterate the take home messages; again, asking students will give you feedback on what has been learnt (but be prepared for some surprises)

Working Effectively and Ethically with Patients

- Think carefully about which parts of the teaching session require direct patient contact; is it necessary to have a discussion at the bedside?
- Always obtain consent from patients before the students arrive
- Ensure that students respect the confidentiality of all information relating to the patient, verbal or written
- Brief the patient before the session; purpose of the teaching session, level of students' experience, how the patient is expected to participate
- If appropriate, involve the patient in the teaching as much as possible
- Ask the patient for feedback; about communication and clinical skills, attitudes, and bedside manner
- Debrief the patient after the session; they may have questions, or sensitive issues may have been raised

Case-Based Teaching

- Case-based teaching inculcates critical thinking and problem solving abilities
- Selection of a case is based upon the goal of the session and learners' prior level of understanding
- Ill-structured cases are more suitable for advanced learners whereas beginners benefit more from simple illustrative cases
- Script for case-based teaching provides direction of learning and brings in structure to the session

Role-Play

- Role-play actively engages the learners and empowers them to take control of their own learning
- Role-play is especially effective in learning counseling and communication skills
- Lack of structure and direction in learning are major barriers that needs to be addressed during role-play
- A script for role-play includes description of content coverage, purpose, problem definition, instructions to role-players and observers
- Teachers' responsibilities in role-play include keeping the play in order, active observation, and feedback

Assessment of Clinical Competence

– Competency is the individual ability to carry out a particular task

– Clinical competency involves amalgamation of many different traits and abilities

– The assessment of clinical competency includes multiple objective tests, valid tools, and direct observation

– Criterion-referenced is the preferred way of interpretation of data from competency assessment

PROBLEM BASED LEARNING (PBL)

Concepts and Rationale

−PBL is an teaching method that challenges the students to "learn to learn", working cooperatively in groups to obtain solutions to real problems

−PBL is a more holistic approach to education; it requires more comprehensive training

−PBL is more likely to meet the needs and demands of medical students, the profession, and society

The PBL Process

– The PBL can be structured as:

  (1) Meeting with the case-writer,

  (2) Helping to form a functioning group, and

  (3) Working and resolution of the case

– Each of the sessions has defined objectives and tutors are responsible to ensure that these objectives are met

– Self-assessment and peer assessment within the group ensure sustainability and progressive growth of the group

Generic Skills and Attitudes

- Teamwork

- Chairing a group

- Listening

- Recording

- Cooperation

- Respect for colleagues' views

- Critical evaluation of literature

- Self directed learning and use of resources

- Presentation skills

Roles of Participants in PBL Tutorial

Scribe

−Record points made by group

−Help group order their thoughts

−Participate in discussion

−Record resources used by group

Tutor

−Encourage all group members to participate

−Assist chair with group dynamics and keeping to time

−Check scribe keeps an accurate record

−Ensure group achieves appropriate learning objectives

−Check understanding

−Assess performance

Chair

−Lead the group through the process

−Encourage all members to participate

−Keep to time

−Ensure group keeps to task in hand

−Ensure scribe can keep up and is making an accurate record

Group Member

- Follow the steps of the process in sequence

- Participate in discussion

- Listen to and respect contributions of others

- Ask open questions

- Research all the learning objectives

- Share information with others

PBL Tutorial Process

Step 1

– Identify and clarify unfamiliar terms presented in the scenario

– Scribe lists those that remain unexplained after discussion

Step 2

– Define the problem or problems to be discussed

– Students may have different views on the issues, but all should be considered

– Scribe records a list of agreed problems

Step 3

– "Brainstorming" session to discuss the problem(s), suggesting possible explanations on basis of prior knowledge

– Students draw on each other's knowledge and identify areas of incomplete knowledge

– Scribe records all discussion

Step 4

– Review steps 2 and 3 and arrange explanations into tentative solutions

– Scribe organises the explanations and restructures if necessary

Step 5

− Formulate learning objectives

− Group reaches consensus on the learning objectives

− Tutor ensures learning objectives are focused, achievable, comprehensive, and appropriate

Step 6

− Private study (all students gather information related to each learning objective)

Step 7

− Group shares results of private study

− Tutor checks learning and may assess the group

Student Assessment in PBL

- Student assessment in PBL should be aligned with the curricular goal
- Students should be assessed on those aspects of knowledge, behaviors, and skills that PBL is supposed to promote
- Besides content knowledge, emphasis should be placed on the students' ability to identify and solve problem, data gathering and interpretation, and application of knowledge in practical situations
- Students should be assessed on their contributions to group process as well

Advantages of PBL

Student Centred

- It fosters active learning, improved understanding, and retention and development of lifelong learning skills

Generic Competencies

- PBL allows students to develop generic skills and attitudes desirable in their future practice

Integration

- PBL facilitates an integrated core curriculum

Motivation

- PBL is fun for students and tutors, and the process requires all students to be engaged in the learning process

"Deep" Learning

- PBL fosters deep learning (students interact with learning materials, relate concepts to everyday activities, and improve their understanding)

Constructivist Approach

- Students activate prior knowledge and build on existing conceptual knowledge frameworks

Disadvantages of PBL

Tutors

– Tutors enjoy passing on their own knowledge and understanding so may find PBL facilitation difficult and frustrating

Human Resources

– More staff have to take part in the tutoring process

Other Resources

– Large numbers of students need access to the same library and computer resources simultaneously

Role Models

– Students may be deprived access to a particular inspirational teacher who in a traditional curriculum would deliver lectures to a large group

Information Overload

– Students may be unsure how much self directed study to do and what information is relevant and useful

Implementation of PBL

- Careful planning and preparation with strong support from academic administrators
- Training of the teachers/tutors/facilitators and students
- Careful design of trigger problems to make them relevant and interesting
- Using language that the students are comfortable with
- Having non-threatening and comfortable surroundings for PBL sessions
- Incorporating on-going group monitoring and evaluation of the PBL process
- Using assessment methods that evaluate the skills obtained from the PBL process

WEB BASED LEARNING

Purpose of Web Based Learning

- Web based learning (E-learning) promises harmonious marriage with learner-centered learning models
- E-learning is supported and delivers multitudes of synchronous and asynchronous learning activities
- E-learning also encourages and promotes collaborative and group learning by creation of virtual community of learners
- Learning objects are smaller and more manageable self-contained components of a large content and one of the preferred methods of curriculum planning in e-learning
- Learning objects are reusable and shareable; they minimize duplication and redundancy in curriculum structures
- The learning material can be linked to libraries, online databases, and electronic journals; particularly useful for research and clinical activities

Features of a Typical Web Based Course

−Course information, notice board, timetable

−Curriculum map

−Teaching materials such as slides, handouts, articles

−Communication via email and discussion boards

−Formative and summative assessments

−Student management tools (records, statistics, student tracking)

−Links to useful internal and external websites—for example, library, online databases, and journals

Advantages of Web Based Learning

−Ability to link resources in many different formats

−Can be an efficient way of delivering course materials

−Resources can be made available from any location and at any time

−Potential for widening access; for example, to part time, mature, or work based students

−Can encourage more independent and active learning

−Can provide a useful source of supplementary materials to conventional programs

Disadvantages of Web Based Learning

- Access to appropriate computer equipment can be a problem for students
- Learners find it frustrating if they cannot access graphics, images, and video clips because of poor equipment
- The necessary infrastructure must be available and affordable
- Information can vary in quality and accuracy, so guidance and signposting is needed
- Students can feel isolated

Advantages of Online Assessment

−Students can receive quick feedback on their performance

−Useful for self assessments; for example, multiple choice questions

−A convenient way for students to submit assessment from remote sites

−Computer marking is an efficient use of staff time

Disadvantages of Online Assessment

– Most online assessment is limited to objective questions

– Security can be an issue

– Difficult to authenticate students' work

– Computer marked assessments tend to be knowledge based and measure surface learning

LEARNING METHODOLOGIES

Concepts and Rationale

- Learner-centered learning is a form of active and reflective learning that is initiated and maintained by the learners' intrinsic motivation to learn
- Group activity and collaboration enhance the learning
- Strategies for learner-centered learning include case-based, project-based, and problem-based learning
- Development of skills for learning is vital for learner-centered learning to be successful
- Surface learning is practiced in situations where motivation for learning is extrinsic. Whereas, in deep learning, the motivation is internal; the desire of the individual to understand and apply what he has learnt
- Experiential learning emphasizes sequential progression of experimentation, observation and reflection, development of general principles, and testing the principles in new situations
- Experiential learning can be applied to improve our own teaching as well as students' learning

Adult Learning

- Adults are independent and self directing
- They prefer learner-centered learning model as this provides greater autonomy and control over their learning
- They have accumulated a great deal of experience, which is a rich resource for learning
- They are more interested in immediate, problem centred approaches than in subject centred ones
- Adults learning is supported by proper utilization of reflective process and development of learning skills
- Life experience is an important determinant of adult learning
- Adults need to feel safe but challenged in a learning situation
- Participatory and group learning are immensely beneficial for adult learners

Self Directed Learning

- Organising teaching and learning so that learning is within the learners' control
- A goal towards which learners strive so that they become able to accept responsibility for their own learning

Self Efficacy - Roles for the Teacher

- Modelling or demonstration
- Setting a clear goal or image of the desired outcome
- Providing basic knowledge and skills needed for the task
- Providing guided practice with corrective feedback
- Giving students the opportunity to reflect on their learning

Constructivism

- The primary idea of constructivism is that learners "construct" their own knowledge on the basis of what they already know
- This theory posits that learning is active, rather than passive, with learners making judgments about when and how to modify their knowledge

Building the Skills of Learning

- "Metacognition" is the skill of learning
- The skill of learning is an important element of learner-centered learning
- At individual learner level, the steps to promote metacognition include helping learner identify the educational needs, developing and implementing a plan, and monitoring and evaluation of the progress

Principles to Guide Learning Process

– The learner should be an active contributor to the educational process

– Learning should closely relate to understanding and solving real life problems

– Learners' current knowledge and experience are critical in new learning situations and need to be taken into account

– Learners should be given the opportunity and support to use self direction in their learning

– Learners should be given opportunities and support for practice, accompanied by self assessment and constructive feedback from teachers and peers

– Learners should be given opportunities to reflect on their practice; this involves analysing and assessing their own performance and developing new perspectives and options

– Use of role models by medical educators has a major impact on learners; medical educators should model these educational principles with theirstudents and junior doctors

STUDENT ASSESSMENT

Concepts and Rationale

– Assessment is an integral component of learning; it is implemented in the context of overall learning and teaching activity

– Good quality assessment not only satisfies the needs of certification but also contributes to students' learning

– It enhances our teaching activities and provides valuable information about the educational processes

– There is a need to implement several changes to make the assessment process more meaningful and in tune with newer learning paradigms

Formative Assessment

– Process-focused

– Collects information from ongoing educational activities and feedbacks to further improve the learning and program effectiveness

– Point of initiation is during the program

– Collects and feedbacks the strengths and weaknesses in order to improve

– Develops knowledge, attitudes, and skills

– Guides and directs towards professional development

– Generally recommended by the professional bodies

Summative Assessment

−Outcome-focused

−Documents the student's achievement or program's worthiness and frequently entails some value judgment

−Point of initiation is generally at the end of program or at a predetermined time (e.g. mid-term examination)

−Records the achievements

−Records existing knowledge, attitudes, and skills

−Summarizes the results of professional development

−Required by the professional bodies

−These two processes are complementary to each other and data from formative assessment are vital for better outcomes during summative assessment

Characteristics of Assessment Instruments

Validity

– The ability of the test to measure what it is supposed to measure

– The two important components are content validity and construct validity

Reliability

– The consistency of the test scores over time, under different testing conditions, and with different raters.

Objectivity

– The degree by which learned and independent examiners agree to the correct answer.

Practicability

– The easiness and feasibility of the test to administer.

Value

– The utility of the test results in producing meaningful conclusions about educational processes.

Validity

- The validity of a test is the extent to which it measures what it purports to measure
- Most competencies cannot be observed directly; therefore, it is important to collect evidence to ensure validity:
- One simple piece of evidence could be, for example, that experts score higher than students on the test
- Alternative approaches include:

    (1) An analysis of the distribution of course topics within test elements (blueprint) and

    (2) An assessment of the soundness of individual test items.

- Good validation of tests should use several different pieces of evidence

Reliability

− A score that a student obtains on a test should indicate the score that this student would obtain in any other given (equally difficult) test in the same field (parallel test)

− A test represents at best a sample selected from a range of possible questions, so if a student passes a particular test one has to be sure that he or she would not have failed a parallel test, and vice versa

− Two factors influence reliability negatively:

(1) Sample error: The number of items may be too small to provide a reproducible result and

(2) Sample too narrow: If the questions focus only on a certain element, the scores cannot generalise to the whole discipline

Choice of Assessment Instruments

- The purpose of assessment should direct the choice of instruments
- Availability, familiarity, and convenience of the instrument should not direct the purpose of the assessment
- Instruments that are highly recommended for one purpose may not necessarily be suitable for other purpose
- No single instrument has all the desired criteria; a reasonable compromise is needed and judgement has to be made
- Instruments for summative assessment should have a high degree of validity and reliability
- Multiple instruments provide a more comprehensive picture than any single instrument

Road Map to Student Assessment

– What is the domain I am interested in assessing?

  Knowledge   Attitude   Skill

– What is the level of competency?

  Knows   Knows how   Apply   Does

– What is the purpose of assessment?

  Formative   Summative

– What is the validity of the instrument for the intended purpose?

  Low   Medium   High

– What is the reliability of the instrument for the intended purpose?

  Low   Medium   High

– Is one instrument sufficient for the purpose?

  Yes   No

WRITTEN ASSESSMENT

Essay Questions and Variations

- Well-written essay questions are good for assessment of higher order cognitive functions such as proposition, synthesis, and evaluation
- The main concerns are relatively low content coverage and relative lack of reliability and consistency in scoring
- Several Short Answer Questions (SAQ) and Modified Essay Questions (MEQ) provide better content coverage and make the scoring easier and more consistent
- Pre-determination of answers and grading criteria is essential before using essay questions as summative assessment tools

Multiple Choice Questions (MCQ) and Variations

– MCQ test knowledge (cognition) but are inefficient in assessing attitudes and skills

– MCQ can assess higher order cognitive functions

– MCQ are favored as they test large content area quickly with a high degree of reliability and consistency

– Incorporation of clinical vignette and integration of basic and clinical science knowledge are recommended in MCQ

– In Extended Matching Item (EMI) the number of options are much higher and include all plausible ones

– EMI offer greater discrimination than limited choice MCQ

– Difficulty and discriminatory indices are used to determine the effectiveness of MCQ and EMI

SKILL BASED ASSESSMENT

Objective Structured Clinical Examination (OSCE)

Planning for OSCE

- Create blueprint

- Set timeline (how long do we need?)

- Get authors for a case-writing workshop

- Review and finalise cases

- Arrange workshop on setting standards

- Recruit standardised patients; recruit faculty members as examiners

- Train standardised patients

- Print marking sheets, make signs

- List all supplies for set-up of OSCE stations

- Remind everyone of date

- Make sure students have all the information

- Plans for the examination day: diagram of station layout; directions for examiners, standardised patients, and staff; possible registration table for students; timing and signals; procedures for ending the examination

Limitations of OSCE

- Stations often require trainees to perform isolated aspects of the clinical encounter, which "deconstructs" the doctor-patient encounter
- OSCE rely on checklists, which tend to emphasise thoroughness; but with increasing experience, thoroughness becomes less relevant
- The limitations on what can be simulated constrain the type of patient problems that can be used

Validity

- Are the patient problems relevant and important to the curriculum?
- Will the stations assess skills that have been taught?
- Have content experts (generalists and specialists) reviewed the stations?

Reliability

- Too few stations or too little testing time
- Checklists or items that don't discriminate (too easy or too hard)
- Unreliable patients or inconsistent portrayals by standardized patients
- Examiners who score idiosyncratically
- Administrative problems (such as disorganised staff or noisy rooms)

Oral Examinations

- Oral examination is useful to assess critical reasoning and problem solving
- Unstructured oral examinations seriously lack the desired level of validity and reliability as a summative assessment tool
- Oral examination is valuable for formative assessment
- Validity and reliability of the oral examination can be improved through faculty education and by instilling proper structure

Standardized Patient

- Standardized patient is a valid and reliable way of assessment of clinical competence
- Standardized patient provides many advantages over traditional paper and pencil based test in clinical competence assessment
- Wide range of acute and chronic, physical and psychological characteristics can be accurately portrayed
- Standardized patient development team is recommended for the successful implementation of standardized patient programs

WORK BASED ASSESSMENT

- The critical factors of portfolio based learning are goal setting, self-reflection, and discovery
- As an educational process it supports self-directed learning, self and collaborative assessment, and progression of personal and professional achievements
- As an assessment instrument, it captures whether the learned knowledge is practiced in real life
- Three aspects of doctors' performance can be assessed:
  (1) Patients' outcomes,
  (2) Process of care, and
  (3) Volume of practice
- Content and organization of portfolio are very much dependent on the primary purpose and educational philosophies behind the development of the portfolio

PROGRAM EVALUATION

Purpose of Evaluation

– To ensure teaching is meeting students' learning needs

– To identify areas where teaching can be improved

– To inform the allocation of faculty resources

– To provide feedback and encouragement for teachers

– To support applications for promotion by teachers

– To identify and articulate what is valued by medical schools

– To facilitate development of the curriculum

Levels of Evaluation

- Teaching program evaluation can be conveniently structured in four levels: reaction, learning, transfer, and results
- Level one assesses the participants' initial reaction to a training program
- Level two assesses the amount of information that learners have learned from the course
- Level three assesses transfer of knowledge, skills or behavior that has been offered in the training program to actual real life
- Level four assesses the ultimate result of the training program
- Each of these levels evaluates specific elements of the program
- An ideal program evaluation planning incorporates elements from each of these levels
- The full impact of the curriculum may not be known until some time after the student has graduated

Kirkpatrick's Four Levels of Evaluation

Level 1

—Learner's reactions

Level 2a

—Modification of attitudes and perceptions

Level 2b

—Acquisition of knowledge and skills

Level 3

—Change in behaviour

Level 4a

—Change in organisational practice

Level 4b

—Benefits to patients or clients

Planning an Evaluation

– What are the goals of the evaluation

– From whom and in what form will data be collected

– Who will collect and analyse data

– What type of analysis, interpretation, and decision rules will be used and by whom

– Who will see the results of the evaluation

Characteristics of an Ideal Evaluation

– Validity

– Reliability

– Acceptability to evaluator and to person being evaluated

– Inexpensiveness

– To reduce possible bias in evaluation, collect views from more than one group; for example, students, teachers, other clinicians, and patients

Participation of Teachers in Evaluation

Self Evaluation

− Academic staff increasingly evaluate their own teaching practice

− Self evaluation is useful if the objective is to provide motivation to change beahviour

− To help define what they are doing, teachers may find it useful to use videotapes made during teaching, logbooks, and personal portfolios

Peer Evaluation

− Direct observation of teachers by their peers can provide an informed, valuable, and diagnostic evaluation

− Mutual classroom exchange visits between trusted colleagues can be valuable to both the teacher and the observer

Participation of Students in Evaluation

−Design: whether the curriculum enables students to reach their learning objectives; whether it fits well with other parts of the curriculum

−Delivery: attributes of teacher and methods used

−Administrative arrangements

Learners Need

−To be involved in developing an evaluation

−To feel their time is respected

−To know their opinions are valued and acted on

Methods of Evaluation

Surveys

− Questionnaires are useful for obtaining information from large numbers of students or teachers about the teaching process.

Interviews

− Individual interviews with students are useful if the information is sensitive

Information from Student Assessment

− Data from assessment are useful for finding out if students have achieved the learning outcomes of a curriculum.

RESEARCH IN MEDICAL EDUCATION

- Research in medical education is generally similar to biomedical research with few notable differences
- Qualitative research is valid and useful in examining new issues, generating range of hypotheses, and proposing newer concepts and premises
- Interventional study with randomization and double-blinding is difficult to achieve in educational research
- Systematic reviews consolidate qualitative or semiquantitative data and effective in dealing with heterogeneous researches
- Need-based research is more feasible and fitting for budding individuals and medical education units

REFERENCES

– Abrahamson S. Essays on medical education. Maryland: University Press of America; 1996.

– Albanese M. Problem-based learning: why curricula are likely to show little effect on knowledge and clinical skills. Medical Education. 2000; 34: 729-38.

– Albanese M, Mitchell S. Problem-based learning: a review of literature on its outcomes and implementation issues. Academic Medicine. 1993; 68: 52-81.

– Amin Z. How do our new graduates prefer to learn? Singapore Medical Journal. 2000; 41: 317-23.

– Anderson B. A snapshot of medical students' education at the beginning of the 21st century: report from 130 schools. Academic Medicine. 2000; 75: 9-12.

– Ashcroft K, Foreman-Peck L. Managing teaching and learning in further and higher education. London: Falmer Press; 1994.

– Barrows H. An overview of the uses of standardized patients for teaching and evaluating clinical skills. Academic Medicine. 1993; 68: 443-53.

– Barrows H. Training standardized patients to have physical findings. Springfield: Southern Illinois University; 1999.

– Bland C, Schmitz D, Stritter F, et al. Successful faculty in academic medicine: essential skills and how to acquire them. New York: Springer; 1990.

– Bligh D. What's the use of lectures? San Francisco: Jossey-Bass; 2000.

– Bligh J, Prideaux D, Parsell G. PRISMS: new educational strategies for medical education. Medical Education. 2001; 35: 520-1.

- Bordage G, Burack J, Irby D, et al. Education in ambulatory settings: developing valid measures of educational outcomes, and other research priorities. Academic Medicine. 1998; 73: 743-50.
- Boud D, Feletti G. The challenge of problem-based learning. 2nd edition. London: Kogan Page; 1998.
- Brazeau C, Crosson J. Changing an existing OSCE to a teaching tool: the making of a teaching OSCE. Academic Medicine. 2002; 77: 932-7.
- Brian J, Lesley R. Medical education in the millennium. Oxford: Oxford University Press; 1998.
- Brinsky A, Dessants B, Flamm M, et al. The art and craft of lecturing. In: Chicago handbook for teachers: a practical guide to the college classroom. Chicago: University of Chicago Press; 1999.
- Brookfield S, Preskill S. Discussion as a way of teaching - tools and techniques for university teachers. Buckingham: Open University Press; 1999.
- Brown G, Manogue M. AMEE medical education guide number 22: refreshing lecturing: a guide for lecturers. Medical Teacher. 2001; 23: 231-44.
- Bruner J. The culture of education. Cambridge: Harvard University Press; 1996.
- Cannon R, Newble D. A handbook for teachers in universities and colleges. 4th edition. London: Kogan Page; 1999.
- Carraccio C, Wolfsthal S, Englander R, et al. Shifting Paradigms: From Flexner to competencies. Academic Medicine. 2002; 77: 361-67.
- Case S, Swanson D. Extended matching items: a practical alternative to free-response questions. Teaching and Learning in Medicine. 1993; 5: 107-115.

References

- Davis M, Harden R. AMEE medical education guide number 15: problem-based learning: a practical guide. Medical Teacher. 1999; 21: 130-40.
- Dent J, Harden R. A practical guide for medical teachers. London: Churchill Livingstone; 2001.
- Duch B, Groh S, Allen D. The power of problem-based learning. Sterling: Stylus; 2001.
- Dyrbye L, Thomas M, Natt N, et al. Prolonged delays for research training in medical school are associated with poorer subsequent clinical knowledge. Journal of Genereal Internal Medicine. 2007; 22: 1101-6.
- Ellaway R, Masters K. e-Learning in medical education Guide 32 Part 1: Learning, teaching and assessment. Medical Teacher. 2008; 30: 455-73.
- Elstein A. Clinical reasoning in medicine. In: Higgs J, Jones M (editors). Clinical reasoning in health professional. Oxford: Butterworth and Heinemann; 1995.
- Eraut M. Developing professional knowledge and competence. London: Falmer; 1994.
- Flexner A. Medical education in the United States and Canada. Carnegie Foundation for the Advancement of Teaching. Bulletin Number 4. New York; 1910.
- Flores-Mateo G, Argimon J. Evidence based practice in postgraduate healthcare education: A systematic review. BMC Health Services Research. 2007; 7: 119-22.
- Forster F, Hounsell D, Thompson S. Tutoring and demonstrating - a handbook. Sheffield: Universities' and Colleges' Staff Development Agency; 1995.
- Forsyth I. Teaching and learning materials and the internet. 3rd edition. London: Kogan Page; 2001.

References

- Furney S, Orsini A, Orsetti K, et al. Teaching the one minute preceptor: a randomized clinical trial. Journal of General Internal Medicine. 2001; 16: 620-4.
- George J, Doto F. A simple five step method for teaching procedural skills. Family Medicine. 2001; 33: 577-8.
- Gwee M, Lee E, Koh D. What is problem-based learning? SMA News. 2001; 33: 6-7.
- Harden R. Twelve tips in organizing an objective structured clinical examination (OSCE). Medical Teacher. 1990; 12: 259-64.
- Harden R. Curriculum mapping: a tool for transparent and authentic teaching and learning. Medical Teacher. 2000; 23: 123-7.
- Harden R, Grant J, Buckley G, et al. BEME Guide No. 1: Best evidence medical education. Medical Teacher. 1999; 21: 553-62.
- Hayes E. Factors that facilitate or hinder mentoring in the preceptor-student relationship. Clin Excell Nurse Pract. 2001; 5: 111-8.
- Hendrie H, Lloyd C. Educating competent and humane physicians. Indianapolis: Indiana University Press; 1990.
- Hutchinson L. Evaluating and researching the effectiveness of educational interventions. British Medical Journal. 1999; 318: 1267-8.
- Irby D. How attending physicians make insructional decisions when conducting teaching rounds. Academic Medicine. 1992; 67: 630-8.
- Irby D. What clinical teacher in medicine needs to know? Academic Medicine. 1994; 69: 333-42.

- Irby D. Three exemplary models of case based teaching. Academic Medicine. 1994; 69: 947-53.
- Jaques D. Learning in groups. 3rd edition. London: Kogan Page; 2000.
- Jolliffe A, Ritter J, Stevens D. The online learning handbook: developing and using web based learning. London: Kogan Page; 2001.
- Jozefowicz R, Koeppen B, Case S, et al. The quality of in-house examinations. Academic Medicine. 2002; 77: 156-61.
- Kaprielian V, Gradison M. Effective use of feedback. Family Medicine. 1998; 30: 406-7.
- Kaufman D, Mann K, Jennett P. Teaching and learning in medical education: how theory can inform practice. London: Association for the Study of Medical Education; 2000.
- Kaufman D, Mann K, Muijtjens A, et al. A comparison of standard-setting procedures for an OSCE in undergraduate medical education. Academic Medicine. 2001; 75: 267-71.
- Kearney R, Puchalski S, Homer Y, et al. The inter-rater and intra-rater reliability of a new Canadian oral examination format in anesthesia is fair to good. Canadian Journal of Anesthesia. 2002; 49: 232-6.
- Kern D, Thomas P, Howard D, et al. Curriculum development for medical education. Baltimore: Johns Hopkins University Press; 1998.
- King A, Perkowski-Rogers L, Pohl H. Planning standardized patient programs: case development, patient training, and costs. Teaching and Learning in Medicine. 1994; 6: 6-14.

References

- Kirkpartick D. Evaluating training programs: the four levels. 2nd edition. Berret Koehler Publisher; 1998.

- Kramer A, Zyuithoff J, Dusman H, et al. Predictive value of a written knowledge test of skills for an OSCE in postgraduate training for general practice. Medical Education. 2002; 36: 812-9.

- Kurtz S, Silverman J, Draper J. Teaching and learning communication skills in medicine. Oxon: Radcliffe Medical Press; 1998.

- Kurtz S, Laidlaw T, Makoul G, et al. Medical education initiatives in communication skill. Cancer Prevention and Control. 1999; 3: 37-45.

- Ludmerer K. Time to heal: American medical education from the turn of the century to the managed care era. New York: Oxford University Press; 1999.

- Marston R, Jones R. Medical education in transition commission on medical education. The sciences of medical practice. Princeton: Robert Wood Johnson Foundation; 1992.

- Masters K, Ellaway R. e-Learning in medical education Guide 32 Part 2: Technology, management and design. Medicl Teacher. 2008; 30: 474-89.

- Mathers N, Challis M, Howe A, et al. Portfolios in continuing medical education - effective and efficient? Medical Education. 1999; 33: 521-30.

- Mayo W, Donnelly M, Schwartz R. Characteristics of the ideal problem-based learning tutor in clinical medicine. Eval Health Prof. 1995; 18: 124-36.

- McGee S, Irby D. Teaching in the outpatient clinic. Journal of General Internal Medicine. 1997; 12: S 34-40.

- Miller G. The assessment of clinical skills, competence, performance. Academic Medicine. 1990; 65: 563-7.
- Neher J, Gordon K, Meyer B, et al. A five-step "Microskills" model of clinical teaching. Journal of the American Board of Family Practice. 1992; 5: 419-24.
- Nendez M, Tekian A. Assessment in problem-based learning in medical schools: a literature review. Teaching and Learning in Medicine. 1999; 11: 323-43.
- Newble D, Cannon R. A handbook for medical teachers. 4th edition. London: Kluwer Academic; 2001.
- Norman G. Research in medical education: three decades of progress. British Medical Journal. 2002; 324: 1560-2.
- Norman G, Schmidt H. Effectiveness of problem-based learning curricula: theory, practice and paper darts. Medical Education. 2000; 34: 721-8.
- Parsell G, Bligh J. Recent perspectives on clinical teaching. Medical Education. 2001; 35: 409-14.
- Paulman P, Susman J, Abboud C. Precepting medical students in the office. London: Johns Hopkins University Press; 2000.
- Pinsky L, Irby D. "If at first you don't succeed": using failure to improve teaching. Academic Medicine. 1997; 72: 973-6.
- Prideaux D. The emperor's new clothes: from objectives to outcomes. Medical Education. 2000; 34: 168-9.
- Print M. Curriculum development and design. Sydney: Allen and Unwin; 1993.
- Reynolds P. Reaffirming professionalism through the education community. Annals of Internal Medicine. 1994; 120: 609-14.

References

- Robson C. Small scale evaluation. London: Sage; 2000.

- Rubenstein W, Talbot Y. Medical teaching in ambulatory care: a practical guide. New York: Springer; 1992.

- Schultheis N. Writing cognitive educational objectives and multiple-choice test questions. American Journal of Health-System Pharmacists. 1998; 55: 2397-401.

- Snell L, Tallett S, Haist S, et al. A review of the evaluation of clinical teaching: new perspectives and challenges. Medical Education. 2000; 34: 862-70.

- Srinivasan M, Wilkes M, Stevenson F, et al. Comparing problem-based learning with case-based learning: effects of a major curricular shift at two institutions. Academic Medicine. 2007; 82: 74-82.

- Stark J. Shaping the college curriculum: academic plans in action. Boston: Allyn and Bacon; 1997.

- Stewart M. Effective physician-patient communication and health outcome: a review. Canadian Medical Association Journal. 1995; 152: 1423-33.

- Sulmasy D. Should medical schools be schools for virtue? Journal of General Internal Medicine. 2000; 15: 514-6.

- Tavanaiepour D, Schwartz P, Loten E. Faculty opinions about a revised pre-clinical curriculum. Medical Education. 2002; 36: 299-302.

- Tiberius R. Small group teaching: a trouble-shooting guide. London: Kogan Page; 1999.

- Towle A. The aims of the curriculum: education for health needs in 2000 and beyond. In: Jolly B, Rees L (editors). Medical Education in the Millennium. New York: Oxford University Press; 1998.

References

- Vernon D, Hosokawa M. Faculty attitudes and opinions about problem-based learning. Academic Medicine. 1996; 71: 1233-8.
- Walberg H, Haertel G. The international encyclopedia of educational evaluation. Oxford; 1990.
- Westberg J, Jason H. Collaborative clinical education: the foundation of effective health care. New York: Springer; 1993.
- Westberg J, Jason H. Fostering learning in the small groups: a practical guide. New York: Springer; 1996.
- WFME Task Force on Defining International Standards in Basic Medical Education. Report of the Working Party. Medical Education, 2000, 34, 665-75.
- Whitcomb M. Competency-based graduate medical education? Of course! But how should competency be assessed. Academic Medicine. 2002; 77: 359-60.
- Whitehouse C, Roland M, Campion P. Teaching medicine in the community: a guide for undergraduate education. New York: Oxford University Press; 1997.
- Wilkes M, Bligh J. Evaluating educational interventions. British Medical Journal. 1999; 318: 1269-72.

www.ingramcontent.com/pod-product-compliance
Lightning Source LLC
Chambersburg PA
CBHW060400190526
45169CB00002B/689